Intermittent Fasting for Women:

The Easy Way to Burn Fat, Feel and Look Good, Slow Ageing and Increase Productivity while Enjoying the Lifestyle and the Foods You Love

Additionally, the information in the following pages is intended only for informational purposes and should thus be thought of as universal. As befitting its nature, it is presented without assurance regarding its prolonged validity or interim quality. Trademarks that are mentioned are done without written consent and can in no way be considered an endorsement from the trademark holder.

Table of Contents

Introduction

Congratulations on downloading the book <u>Intermittent Fasting For Women</u> and thank you for taking the initiative to do so. This is a great step towards achieving the lifestyle that you ultimately desire! The following chapters discuss the causes of obesity, what intermittent fasting is, and how this time tested method can help you achieve your goals for weight loss, mental productivity, and optimal health. You'll enjoy the step-by-step tutorial for starting and maintaining the intermittent fasting diet.

This is the book you need if you are looking for a way to give yourself the foundation and instruction to change your health for the better. Intermittent fasting places awareness and control in your hands to decide when, what, and how much you need to eat. You can finally break free of the bondage of breakfast, lunch, and dinner routines that pack unwanted and unnecessary calories into your body.

The practice of intermittent fasting helps you develop a healthier relationship with food and increases your ability to rethink current eating patterns. Put an end to negative eating habits, develop a healthy eating style, and become fit, alert and better equipped to deal with whatever situation life brings your way. When you are finished reading this book, you'll know what intermittent fasting is and the numerous health and lifestyle benefits it offers.

If you are a woman, you have chosen the right book. This particular book contains information and resources that are specifically meant for women. The information included is all written with this approach in mind, by a woman who understands that women metabolize and process foods differently than men and that women's bodies respond to different stimuli and different environmental stressors. It is not appropriate to use the same fasting approach for men and women any more than it would be appropriate for them to wear the same clothing or choose the same vitamin supplements.

This book lays out the background and basics women need to understand the process of intermittent fasting, what the requirements are, and what the method entails. It also provides specifics on eating plans, schedules and other details to help you find the right approach that works best for you.

Have you experimented with intermittent fasting in the past and had a negative or less than ideal experience? This book will give you a whole new perspective. You'll learn real strategies you can start right away. You can design your own personal pathway to ultimate health and wellness. Learn to transition slowly, get comfortable with the routine and even continue with regular exercise!

Fasting, much like a low-carbohydrate and high-fat diet, is an additional dietary way to increase weight loss, along with the addition of a few other health benefits. Long-term use will be required to see the most benefits when it comes to leaning out and losing considerable amounts of body fat.

This book provides the basics on how to use intermittent fasting as a tool to your greatest possible benefit. Here are some positive points about intermittent fasting that will be covered in depth in this book:

- Most women find it easier to follow than other diets because you simply bypass meals, which is uncomplicated when you're stretched for time or not hungry.
- You can fit intermittent fasting into any lifestyle. Customize it to fit special occasions like birthdays or holidays.
- You develop the technique that's right for you to control hunger and discovering more about *why, when and how* you turn to food.

Every effort was made to ensure this book is full of as much useful information as possible. Please do enjoy!

Chapter 1: The Basics

Why are we so fat?

The root cause of obesity is receiving more energy from the foods eaten than the body burns before refueling with even more food. Current research findings align on this fundamental point: weight management, energy metabolism, physical activity, and behavior are inextricably linked. The lives that most of us lead do not provide for a healthy lifestyle that balances our energy requirements with our metabolic activity.

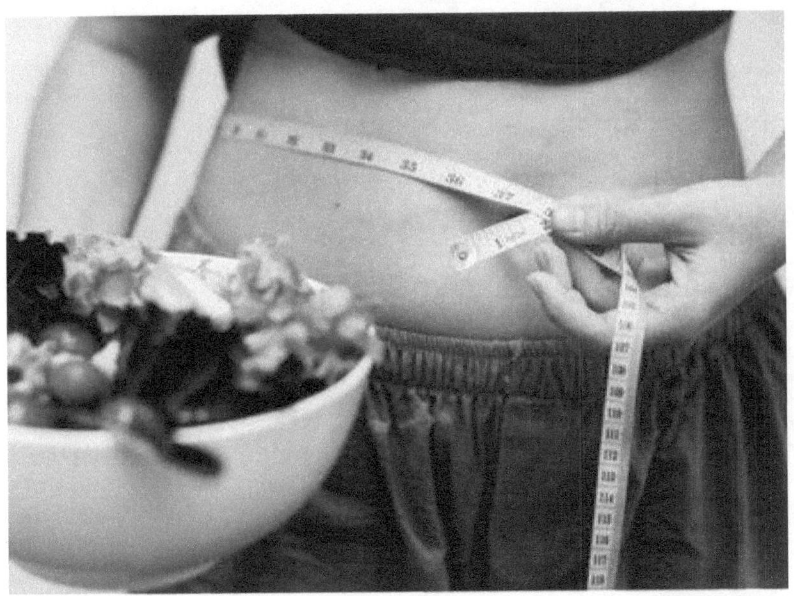

This energy balance framework is a powerful concept in understanding the regulation of body weight. Recent evidence favors the idea that food intake is more important than altering energy expenditure. This means, simply put, that the most important step you can take towards achieving weight loss goals is to alter eating habits. There is no time like the present to initiate this process and start building a better way of eating and living.

What is Intermittent Fasting?

The idea of fasting is not new in any way. In fact, it's an ancient practice that has existed in many forms and evolved over time in a variety of cultural contexts. When discussing fasting, it's important to differentiate between an absolute or dry fast. The difference is referring to abstaining from all food or eliminating liquids for a specified period. Dry fasting is typically done over a prolonged period.

Fasting can also be defined as the willing abstinence from some food, drink, or both, for a set time. Since the beginning of the earliest human societies, people have lived through periods of nutritional hardship. It varied from short to long amounts of time with minimal sustenance, to the extremes of no food at all. This history of hardship and deprivation can understandably associate fasting with a dire and desperate situation. It might be valid in some instances, but it does not provide a complete picture.

Starting at the beginning of human societies, there have always been spiritual practices that either benefited from or required fasting. Many of these have influenced some of the cleansing and dieting philosophies that still exist today. One of the modern programs that have risen and fallen in popularity is called the Master Cleanse, or lemonade diet. It's traditionally a 14-day diet that consists of lemonade made with cayenne pepper and maple syrup. Although there may be great benefits to be had from following this diet, it's never gone mainstream. It's not easy for a woman to maintain heavy work commitments, children to care for, or other time constraints.

Perhaps it would be a stretch to say there is widespread acceptance of fasting, but there have been subcultures that long promoted the practice in some form or another. Up until now, most fasting regimes have tended to be difficult and not that much fun. This has changed with the rise of intermittent fasting. It's a practice assessable to working women because it doesn't require you to withdraw from daily life and activities. It's perfectly possible to undertake an intermittent fasting program while you are working, exercising and doing whatever else you do on a *normal daily basis.*

There are many different types of intermittent fasting, such as the 16/8 or 5:2 regimen. At a minimum, intermittent fasting involves a brief cessation of calories of 12-16 hours, generally during the night time hours. Most of us are fasting overnight between dinner and breakfast anyway, but intermittent fasting is more specific. Some people eat only during an eight-hour window during the day, while some take a whole 24-hour fast.

In general, a 24-hour fast is not appropriate for most women. More details on the possible methods will be discussed in detail in Chapter 2. Whatever timeframe is chosen, the practice of intermittent fasting is possible to incorporate into daily life because it involves *fasting that occurs at irregular intervals* that are set by the individual and designed according to her preference.

This is the revolutionary secret of intermittent fasting: it can be tailored to the individual woman, rather than requiring her to conform to an extreme or unrealistic regime. This makes it fun and adaptable! You set the rules according to a plan that works for you.

Why Should I Use Intermittent Fasting?

While fasting, the body does not remain in a passive state. It might appear that the body is in a calm state of stasis, but that's far from the case. Intermittent fasting is an exercise strategy that strengthens the capacity of metabolism to burn fat. The parallels between intermittent fasting and exercise are numerous. Fasting induces a metabolic workout that accomplishes all the following:

- Decreases measurable blood sugar
- Reduces insulin levels
- Mobilizes lipids and fatty acids
- Increases fat oxidation
- Promotes weight loss and makes it easier to stay at a healthy weight
- Balances hormones and revs up your fat burning potential
- Reduces swelling and pain in the body
- Helps prevent diabetes type 2
- Markedly reduce your chances of heart disease

Sound familiar? Without going to the gym or going for a jog, you are receiving similar benefits to those you'd receive from exercising. The time you spend not eating is referred to as "the

fasted state". The time during the day you eat is referred to as the **"fed"** state. **While** in the **fasted** state, (rather than the **fed** state), the body rapidly and efficiently mobilizes free fatty acids from adipose stores (a fancy name for fat tissue).

Practicing intermittent fasting helps strengthen our bodies to burn fat in contrast with our more common **fed** state. The body during the fed state relies on frequent resupplies of glucose and sugar for fuel. In addition to weight loss, stimulating and strengthening the metabolism provides numerous other health benefits that include enhanced mental clarity, focus, and stress reduction. The process and practice of intermittent fasting sharpens the mind and neural functions while reshaping the physical structure of our bodies at the cellular and molecular levels.

Health & Lifestyle Benefits of Intermittent Fasting

One of the most exciting applications of intermittent fasting may be its ability to slow the process of aging. It allows the body to regenerate naturally, which, over time, slows the breaking down processes that contribute to aging. It's also shown promise to improving memory loss and lessens other symptoms associated with dementia. There's no cure for dementia, but preventative measures can alleviate early stages, or decrease the potential for early onset of this devastating condition.

The effect of intermittent fasting on the aging process is partially credited to the fact that this dietary change is good for our brains at any stage of life. It changes the chemistry and function of our cells, genes, and hormones. While in the **fasted** state, our bodies initiate important cellular repair processes and hormone level shifts. These naturally occurring regenerative processes are allowed to function at their full potential because we're giving our bodies a much-needed break from processing food. These regenerative processes also contribute to improved mental health and psychological well-being. Below are some of the health benefits that occur during fasting:

- Human growth hormone: The blood levels of growth hormones may increase as much as 5-fold during the **fasted** state. Higher levels of this hormone enhance fat burning and muscle gain.
- Cellular repair: The body naturally enters an active state where waste materials are removed from cells. Cells also initiate important processes that can change our genetic responses.

- Gene expression: Beneficial changes in gene expression and molecules take place which helps build immunity and protection against disease.

- Enhanced hormone function & lower insulin levels: This state allows for the breakdown of body fat. This is the exact process that serves to facilitate weight loss. According to a 2014 literature review, there is scientific evidence that intermittent fasting can cause weight loss of 3-8% of total body weight in just 3 weeks to 2 months.

In addition to all the benefits listed above, intermittent fasting has the added benefit of speeding the process of fat loss in the abdominal area, which is one of the hardest places for women to achieve their ideal body shape. Not only can it help women get rid of belly fat, but it also decreases the risks of disease by reducing harmful stores of fat.

And, last, but not least, this dietary plan can save time in the kitchen since there are fewer meals to plan for and prepare. Who wouldn't want time away from kitchen duty?

Intermittent Fasting for Women

There are special considerations to be taken for women considering trying intermittent fasting. Though intermittent fasting can be a simple, convenient, and effective way to lose weight, care must be taken to follow an approach that works with the natural processes of the body. Carelessly entering and exiting this type of dietary change can work against your natural body functions. Female bodies are extremely sensitive to calorie reduction and blood sugar level changes.

When the caloric intake and blood sugar levels are low in women, hormone secretion processes may be disrupted. This can have far-reaching effects on women, leading to shifts in mood, menstrual cycles, and poor bone health under more extreme instances. What this means is that women need to follow a modified approach to intermittent fasting.

Initially, it's very important for women new to intermittent fasting to include shorter fasting periods and fewer fasting days. This can be modified over time to incorporate longer fasting periods as the body adjusts, but it's important to make this a gradual process.

Why Intermittent Fasting is Different for Men and Women

Men Respond Well – All the Time

When a well-matched group of men and women set out to stick with an intermittent fasting dietary regime, the results are a little different and come down in the favor of men. Males that follow the routines to the letter show a 100 percent success rate. Women lag a little behind with a 99 percent success rate. The difference can be as subtle as the emotional levels of women that vary during the month and the degree of stress and anxiety-impact of critical life events.

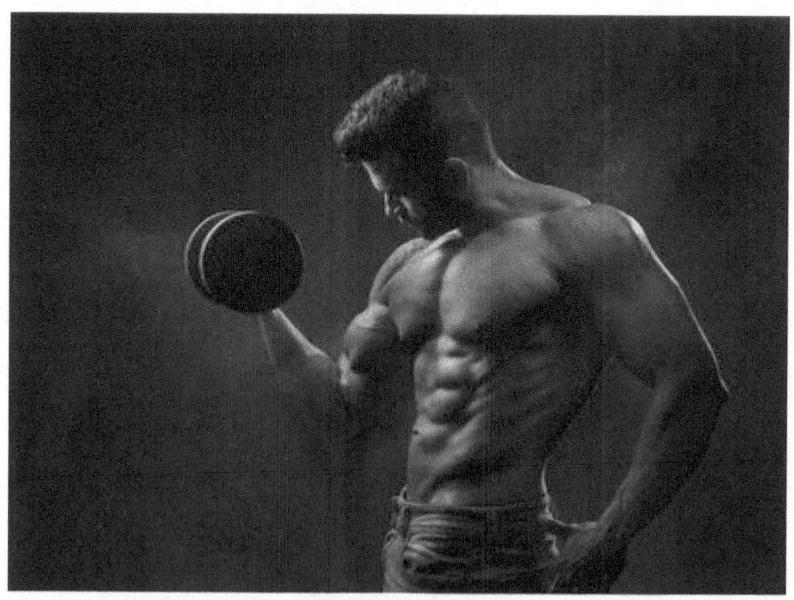

It doesn't mean that men are not affected in some ways, but women seem to suffer more from sluggish metabolism during periods of high stress and tension. The good news is that 99 percent of women do find that intermittent fasting brings them the positive results they desire. Rather than turning yourself into a statistic, try and prepare for the fasting process ahead of time and you should see good results.

Emotional Control and Triggers

Emotions can exercise more than ample control over your daily activities. It can lead to binge eating, snacking out of boredom, or being upset. It can lower your levels of daily activity and create a sluggish metabolic rate. It's these times in combination that seem to allow everything you eat to go to your waistline. Women struggle more with emotional controls due to the close connection that is naturally inherent in nurturing behaviors. You don't have to be a parent to feel nurturing instincts.

Your best defense against moments of emotions that cloud the progress you make is to understand your personal triggers. Be aware of the times and situations that can set you back and off-track on your intermittent fasting routine. The better you are on guard, the less likely you will fall victim to emotional eating and falling off the fasting wagon.

Body Size Differences and Sensitivities

The sheer size difference between most men and women make it abundantly clear that the response to intermittent fasting will be far different between the two. Men are absolute powerhouses of energy and fuel that can breeze through a 16 or 18-hour fast with hardly a whimper. Women should slowly work up to this and can still be completely wiped out after an extended-hours fast. Much of the reason men seem so unfazed is the fact there is a larger body mass to draw from in reserves of energy.

Women tend to be more sensitive to the slightest changes in blood sugar levels. You could feel perfectly fine one day during an intermittent fast and get dizzy and disoriented the next. You may have to take a closer look as to the quality of your diet between fasting periods and whether you are taking in enough water. Either problem can leave you weak and dizzy.

Think Long-Term

Women should set long-term goals when it comes to intermittent fasting. Trying to achieve success within a few weeks is not a reasonable amount of time for women. Progress should be made slow and steady to ensure its safe. Only move along in intensity and longer fasting periods when you feel you have completely mastered the level you are on. Any sense of physical discomfort or mental distress should have you draw back a step before moving forward. You won't lose anything by being safe.

Instead of hoping for dramatic results in six-weeks, plan for revisiting your progress in six months, or even a year. Intermittent fasting is a much more productive way of improving health and maintaining a healthy weight by creating a long-term lifestyle around the program. Fasting of this type is like weight loss in general. It's the long-term loss that counts as permanent. Anyone can drop a few pounds for a week or two, but is the drop real weight loss, or simply dehydrating yourself? Plan a steady pace that moves you forward at a comfortable rate.

Forgive the Slips and Get Back on Track

Don't fall into the trap of losing motivation if you make a slip or two and end a fasting period early. If this happens, wait it out and try again. Explore the reasons behind the slip. Trying to continue with a fast when going to events that are serving all sorts of tempting foods can be problematic. It can be difficult to explain to family or friends that you're partaking in a fast and a slip happens. In order to avoid limitations to your lifestyle try to schedule these events with **fed** periods and do **fasting** periods when you are not going to eat out.

Illness can also account for times that a fasting period has to be cut short. Even a slight head cold can throw off your metabolism and require that eat three square meals a day until it clears. Sudden increases in physical demands on the body can also throw you off a fast. Without realizing it, work or home demand can suddenly increase the number of calories you need to feel comfortable moving around. If you feel ravenously hungry, discontinue the fasting period and eat healthy and nutritious foods. Deprivation will make you begin to dread and dislike intermittent fasting.

How to Prepare for Intermittent Fasting

Good preparation is the best way to enter an intermittent fasting routine with a positive attitude and a healthy body. Taking care of nutrition and hydration before it becomes a serious problem is your best defense against having to stop and start all over again.

Skip a Major Meal

Is the thought of experiencing tremendous amounts of hunger pains holding you back from trying intermittent fasting? Choose from missing out completely on breakfast, lunch, or dinner. Make it the primary meal you eat of the day. Eat no snacks between the meal before and after the one you miss. It will give you an idea of what the hunger pains are like at their worst.

Do this every other day, three times a week to prepare for the upcoming start of your first fasting period. Combined with logging your current eating habits and making some nutritional changes, the practice will serve you well towards succeeding. You should no longer dread the first portion of fasting, which is getting comfortable with a periodically empty stomach.

Concentrate on Hydrating Well Beforehand

Water will be your best friend during an intermittent fast. It helps pump up your metabolism and keeps your engines running smooth, no matter how lean you are on fuel. Adjust your water intake to the level that is comfortable and healthy for you. Do this for at least a month before starting your first fasting period. It helps ensure you are not starting from a place of possible dehydration.

Eating the recommended amounts of fruits and vegetables daily will also be a great way to get and stay hydrated. You will also benefit tremendously from the infusion of natural vitamins and minerals. Keep plenty of healthy snack items on hand for the times you do have to end a fasting period early. At least you will have healthy foods to fall back on.

Begin Eating a Good Diet of Nutritious Foods and Snacks

Although people enjoy benefits of intermittent fasting without changing their diet, intermittent wasting in combination with healthier foods will help you to achieve your goals more faster. Take every bit of processed foods in your house and toss them out before starting your fasting. Foods that are chemically loaded, high in sugars, and processed into empty-calorie junk are no good for anyone. It's the best time to completely make a sweeping change in your eating habits that will benefit you your entire life.

Reducing the bad foods and introducing healthy items are what will help lower your chances for cancer, diabetes, heart attacks, strokes, and all sorts of maladies. The change in diet alone will literally add years to your life. Healthy eating will also help keep your focus on a healthier lifestyle as the reason behind the intermittent fasting. Focus will be critical on days that seem hard to get through. No matter how well you plan, you will experience a day or two that is a struggle.

End After-Dinner and Midnight Snacking

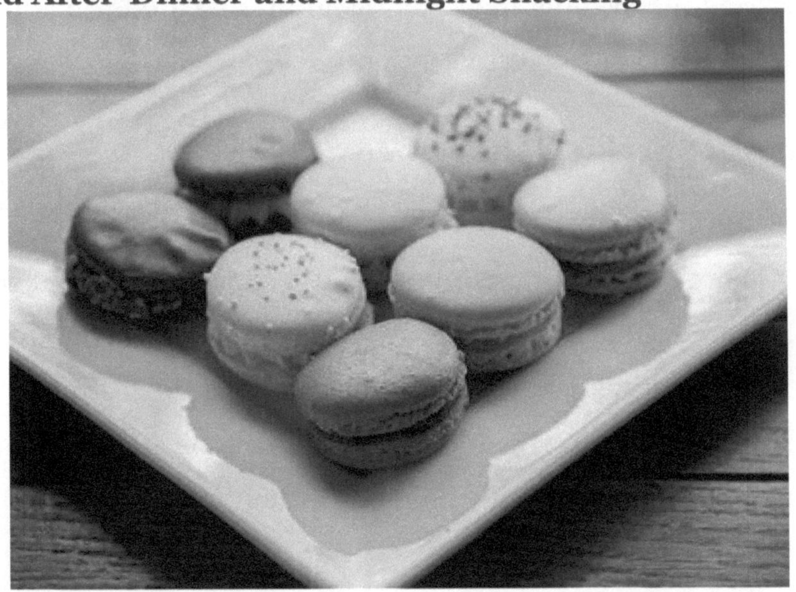

Snacking, no matter how slight or healthy the item, is a break in the chain during your fasting period. It's far better to train yourself before starting to cut out after-dinner and late-night or midnight snacks. You can do this by gradually switching over to healthier foods, but eventually cut it out completely. Do your snacking during the morning hours and daylight times. It becomes comfortable faster than you might think.

Much of the struggles with intermittent fasting are due to the bad eating habits developed over a lifetime. Break these bad habits before you even start the first fasting period. You will give yourself a boost in success without even trying. If you have always been big on a heavy evening snack, you might find that you sleep better by keeping your stomach concentrated on digesting the evening meal. Piling additional foods on adds to the stress on your digestive system.

Cut Out Snacking Altogether

Wait until you are about two weeks away from starting your first fasting period and completely cut snacks from your diet. Focus on eating healthy, nutritious meals only. You can go back to snacking healthy items once starting the fasting at the appropriate times. The addition of extra food items at times will then seem like you are being rewarded, rather than feeling instantly deprived.

Intermittent fasting is a good way to cleanse the body and get it to a state of optimal operation. Food deprivation thoughts can be a huge hindrance in your ability to stick with a routine fasting schedule. The elimination of snacks completely and sudden reappearance at appropriate times is a simple way to relax the mind away from thoughts that the body is being unnecessarily deprived of nutrition. Your odds of success climb exponentially.

Stay in Tune with Your Body

Take all the time you need to prepare to start your first fasting period. Your body will let you know when you are as ready as you can be. Nothing can truly prepare you for the total experience if you've never fasted for long periods before. Understand that it will be some time in the future before you are attempting fasts that exceed 12-hours in duration. Nearly everyone has had to go 12-hours without food at some time or another.

Never start a fasting period without feeling fully confident you are healthy and in a good mental place for the duration. High holiday times and stressful scheduled events are the wrong time to pile more on your plate. Go with the flow and you'll find the right time and date comes up naturally. Make the planning as stress-free as the experience. Focus on how much healthier you will feel at this same time next year.

Who Should Not Fast?

If you have a history of eating disorders, hypoglycemia, adrenal fatigue or hypothyroidism, intermittent fasting is not appropriate for you.

If you have ever had, or suspect you may have an eating disorder, do not take on intermittent fasting. It's appropriate to seek care from a professional and find a different program that works for your unique needs.

Even though you may want to consider intermittent fasting as a method for achieving your ideal weight (18.5 – 24.9 BMI), it's not appropriate for those who are underweight (below 18.5 BMI). Your BMI (Body Mass Index) can indicate if you are normal weight and is calculated using formula below.

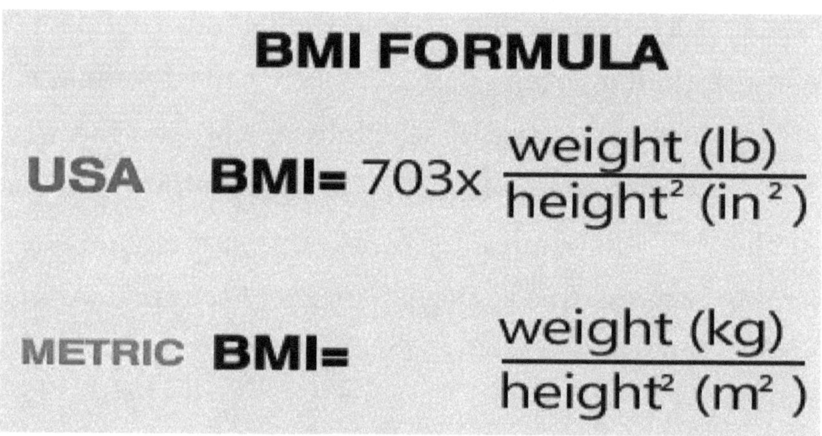

Women who are pregnant, trying to become pregnant, actively breastfeeding, or who have had trouble conceiving should also steer clear of intermittent fasting. Intermittent fasting is known to change hormonal levels and alter body chemistry. It can also have an impact on menstrual cycles or breast milk production.

While fasting is not appropriate during pregnancy or post-partum, there are variations and companion eating styles that work with less hormonal disruption. For example, it's not only safe to increase healthy fats and restrict refined and processed grains during pregnancy and while breastfeeding – it's strongly suggested. It will benefit both mother and baby! A carefully designed, low-carbohydrate, high-fat diet has been proven to help pregnant women in general, especially those that are diagnosed with gestational diabetes. This example drives home just how safe and therapeutic these companion diets can be.

Chapter 2: How To Do Intermittent Fasting

Main Strategies for Fasting for Women

The best approach for most women embarking on the intermittent fasting lifestyle is to start with shorter periods of time in the **fasted** state and modify as the individual's body chemistry and health permits. The safest approach is to start with less time in the **fasted** state. It's important to gauge health and fitness and make careful observations before increasing this time period.

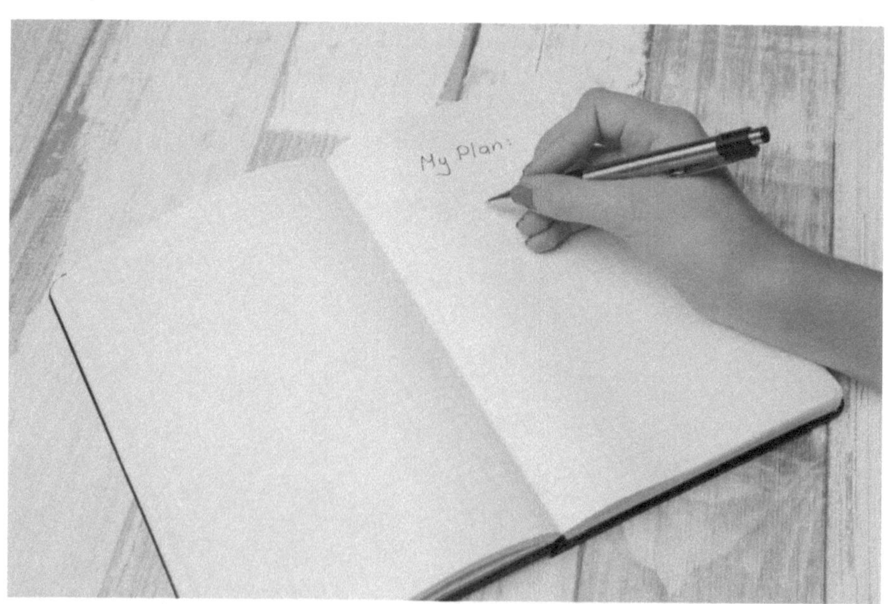

Everybody is unique and each person will respond slightly differently as the beneficial regenerative processes triggered by intermittent fasting begin to take effect. Generally, given adequate time to adapt, many women can spend increasing amounts of time in the **fasted** state. There are four popular ways for women to safely do intermittent fasting. These are listed below according to the total time spent in the **fasted** state.

- *Alternate-day:* Spend 14-16 hours every other day in the **fasted** state
- *14/12 routine:* Spend 12 hours in the **fasted** state each day
- *16/8 routine:* Spend 16 hours in the **fasted** state each day
- *5/2 routine:* Spend 2 days each week in the **fasted** state

Another popular routine of intermittent fasting is called the *Warrior diet.* It's where a woman typically eats one large meal during a 24-hour period. This method is only suitable for women who wish to alter or control estrogen levels, but it may also be a safe method only for an experienced intermittent faster.

Which Type of Intermittent Fasting is Best for You?

Most women will benefit from a slow, steady approach to intermittent fasting. This can easily be initiated by gradually increasing the period of time between dinner and breakfast you eat the following morning. Spending just 2 additional hours in the fasted state every 24-hours, one or more times per week, is a perfect place to start. This requires no conscious effort beyond setting a time for dinner and breakfast and eating no food at night between the designated meal times. See below for an example of a beginning intermittent fasting diet:

8:00 AM: Breakfast
12:30 PM: Lunch
5:00 PM: Dinner
Nothing is eaten until 7:00-8:00 AM for the next day's breakfast.
*(14-15 hour interval in the **fasted** state)*

Once you have taken this first step, you'll be well on the way to consciously changing your eating patterns. It's appropriate to add days with a 14-hour **fasted** period as much as feels right for your body. For some women who already regularly spend 14 or more hours without eating, it may be appropriate to begin with a 16-hour fasting interval one or more days per week. See below for an example of a daily program:

10:00 AM: Breakfast
2:00 PM: Lunch
6:00 PM: Dinner
No food eaten until 10:00 AM for the next day's breakfast.
(*16-hour interval in the **fasted** state*)

Some women may want to dive in with the 16/8 approach and spend 16 hours per day in the **fasted** state every day to achieve their health goals. This is only appropriate for women who are healthy, fit and with no extenuating circumstances that might impact body functions on the metabolic level. The 16/8 method equates to over 100 hrs/week in the **fasted** state and that's the maximum amount of time recommended for any woman new to intermittent fasting. It may be appropriate to add even more hours *after your body has had time to adjust.*

For many women, it's appropriate to build in some 18-hour periods in the **fasted** state once given time to acclimate to the lifestyle of intermittent fasting. The beauty of intermittent fasting is that you decide how long you want the fasting period to be, and what span of time you want to eat within. Fasting can be tailored to your lifestyle as you deem fit. You can begin your eating period at 7 am and end it at 5 pm. You'll still reap benefits from intermittent fasting. Alternatively, you could start it at 11 am, and end it at 9 pm and receive the identical benefits.

With good results, you could slowly increase the number of days during the week that you follow the plan. And, ultimately, given a positive response from your body, you could gradually increase the fasting period during the days you follow intermittent fasting. How the process unfolds is up to you, your individual body, and unique life situation. In summary, keep the following guidelines in mind:

- A maximum of 14-hours in the **fasted** state is initially recommended.
- Start with 1-2 days/week and gradually build on that.
- Do not fast on consecutive days during your first 2-3 weeks of fasting (for instance, if you do a 16-hour fast, do it on Wednesday or Friday & Sunday rather than on Monday, Tuesday and Wednesday).
- It is best to find a consistent program that works for your body and lifestyle.
- Spending any more than 24-hours fasting *at an absolute maximum* is not recommended.

Chapter 3: Intermittent Fasting for Weight Loss

Learn About Your Natural Eating Pattern

The first step towards any change in diet is awareness. Start paying attention to what you're eating and begin being conscious of your dietary choices. This will serve you well during the **fed** periods of your intermittent fast. It's a well-known fact that one of the best ways to change unhealthy eating habits is to first document the foods you eat, when, and how much.

The best way to keep track of them is to write them down in a small notebook. Carry a pen and paper or make notes in an app on your phone or tablet about when and what you eat. Most people are shocked by how much they eat in a day. Identifying personal eating patterns and the types of foods preferred is the appropriate place to start when embarking on intermittent fasting.

Create a food journal or log (you will find a link in bonus section to get a copy of a free printable food journal) that includes the following items:

- *Log the Date and day of the week*: Note whether it's morning, noon, or night. You'll have to be time-specific when you start fasting.

- *What are all the foods and drinks consumed*: List the types, amounts, and whether you added calories through use of condiments, butter, sugar, etc. Beverages count, so make note of them too. Keep notes on what you add to your beverages, such as sugar or honey as a sweetener. This will be important later.

- *Portion sizes*: Estimates of the volume, weight or number of items works just fine. If you prefer to measure, that's great as well. The point is to get a sense of quantity.

- *The location of your meals*: Take notes of where you are at mealtimes. Are you in a car, at a desk, or on a couch? Are you eating alone or with other people?

- *What is your activity level while eating*: Pay attention to what you are focused on as you're eating food. Are you browsing the internet or checking Instagram, or simply talking with friends?

- *How are you feeling*: What are your emotions? Are you happy, excited, depressed, stressed, anxious, or content? Our emotions can direct our eating choices, and conversely, eating can inspire emotions. Pay particular attention to increases in eating based on emotional situations.

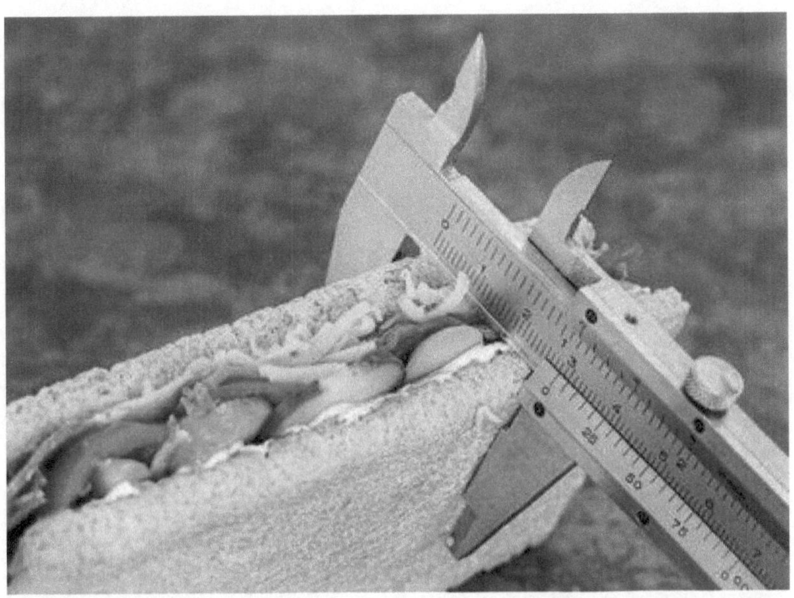

To make your food journal valuable, be open and honest. Take the time to note every bite of food eaten and beverage you drink. If you don't log everything, you won't have an accurate picture of your dietary habits. For the most accurate results, try to record your food intake within 15-minutes of the time you eat.

Use a daily food journal for 7-days. They don't have to be consecutive days. The goal is just to get an illustration of what your natural tendencies and preferences are with foods. This will provide the information you need later about your habits and serve the purpose of acclimating your mind to the task of being aware of what you eat, when, why, and how you feel.

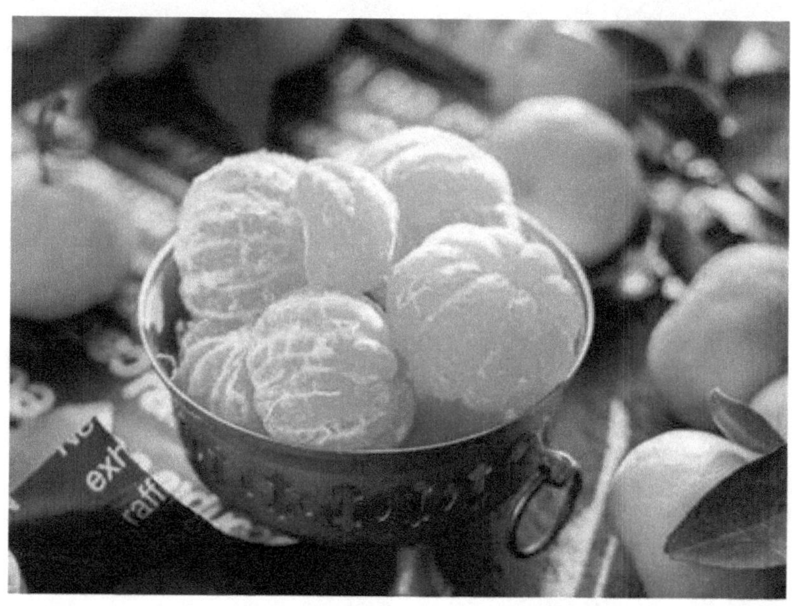

It's not fundamental that you eat a perfectly balanced diet, but good choices will serve you well. There are entire books written on what is best to eat. Try to eat a well-balanced diet that includes plenty of whole grains, vegetables, fruits, and proteins. Try to limit processed foods and sugar. Include healthy fats like those found in olive oil, nuts, avocados and whole milk products for beneficial nutrients. See the chart below for an example of a healthy daily eating guide.

MY DAILY HEALTHY EATING GUIDE

Food	Serves per day	Sample serving size
Breads, cereal, rice, pasta, noodles	4-6	2 slices bread, 1 bread roll, 1 cup rice
Vegetables	5	1/2 cup cooked vegetables, 1 cup salad vegetables, 1 small potato
Fruit	2	1 medium piece of fruit, 2 smaller pieces of fruit, 1 cup diced or canned fruit
Milk, yoghurt, cheese	2-3	1 (250 milk) cup milk, 200g yoghurt, 1 cup soy milk (calcium fortified), 40g cheese. Choose low fat varieties.
Meat, fish, eggs, nuts, legumes	1-1.5	65-100g lean meat, or 80-120g cooked fish (1small fillet), or 1/2 cup dried beans or lentils, 1/3 cup peanuts or almonds, 1/4 cup seeds
Extra foods	0-2.5	2 Biscuits, 1 glass alcohol, a little chocolate, jam or honey, 1 tablespoon oils and fats

Start with an Easier Fast

It's important to pace yourself and begin with shorter duration fasts for multiple reasons. Your body needs time to adjust. Fasting is hard work. All you need to do is put in the initial effort to re-structure an eating schedule and the natural processes of the body will take it from there. The fact that the process is happening out of sight means you need to value it even more. Your metabolism will be working overtime. The fabric and tissues that make up your body will be undergoing a transformation at the cellular level. It's critical you don't underestimate the efforts required to fuel the regenerative processes your body will undertake.

Don't make it impossibly hard by diving in with a marathon approach and fasting for 18-hours, every day of the week. It's much better to ease into the process with a 14-hour fast, 2-3 days/week. This will give your body time to acclimate to a new state, and you will be much less likely to experience hunger pains, cravings, or unpleasant side effects, such as fatigue or headaches.

Keep the intermittent fasting process simple from the beginning. Plan to consume only water, black coffee, or unsweetened tea when fasting. While eating, don't worry too much about your diet, or achieving the perfect combination of foods right away. Focus more on completing the fast and adjusting the times as needed to suit your schedule. Remember to stick to the time period you set for the **fasted** state.

When you choose a specific day you'd like to fast on, pick one you are likely to say "Where did all the time go?" or, "The day got away from me!" If your mind is on other things, you are less likely to focus on the difficulty of fasting. You're more likely to finish your fast successfully. If you slip up, forgive yourself. This is not a high-stakes diet. It's a process about getting to know yourself and your eating habits. Get yourself back on track and pick up wherever you left off. Try the plan outlined below for an easy, no risk intermittent fasting plan that's safe for most healthy women that are beginners.

Day 1: *Eat dinner at 7 pm.* The hard part will be not eating anything after dinner. You may feel hungry, but it's unlikely you really are if its 8-9pm and you just had a good meal at 7 pm. The evening is the time of the day when you are most likely to be at home, either unwinding or moving your way through your weekly routine. If snacking is part of that, this may be a challenging time to take your mind off popcorn, chips, or ice cream. Remind yourself why you are fasting and think about all the benefits you can get while watching a movie, reading a book, or preparing for the next day. Enjoy some tea or a glass of water and assure yourself this is the very hardest part of your fast. Once the evening is over and you get into bed, you just need a way to relax and enjoy the rest of the night. Time flies when you are sleeping.

Day 2: *Delay eating breakfast.* Take the time to celebrate the fact you just did a 12-hour fast. The longer you can delay breakfast, the better. You only need to wait until 9 am. That's it! If you're heading to work, think about something you could bring with you or pick up on the way, such as fruit and yogurt, or a power smoothie. Prepare or bring something you'll really enjoy eating because you deserve it. For some people, morning rush time at 7 is not an ideal time to eat. If this is you, capitalize on it. Don't just grab a banana or a piece of toast to eat in the car. Bring water, tea, or coffee with you if you are leaving, or enjoy a cup wherever you are. (Be careful with coffee- it does not agree with everyone on an empty stomach.) There is nothing all that unusual about waiting to have your first meal of the day when it's convenient. You may have to wait until the house is empty, a few chores are done, and you clear some time to sit and enjoy the rest of the morning. The point is that there is no rush. If you stay busy, you might not even be thinking about the fast.

9:30-10 AM: Time for breakfast! Take a break and enjoy it if you can. At noon, you probably won't be hungry yet because you just ate a couple of hours ago. No need to make yourself eat just because it's lunch time!

2:00 PM: Lunch. You are probably hungry by now, but you've had a nice block of time to accomplish something in the meantime. Have a nice lunch.

Serve dinner by 7 PM: Build up on the prior steps: No eating afterward but eat breakfast at a normal time the next morning. Take a 12-hour break this time.

<u>**Day 3:**</u> *Eat breakfast at 7 AM* and have lunch at noon or 1 PM, *unless you are not hungry until later.* Pay attention to what your body needs, but remember, don't snack. Have water, coffee or tea instead.

Wait a few days and repeat this program. This is a simple, no risk way to begin intermittent fasting. Follow this method for the first 2-3 weeks to give your body time to adapt.

Intermittent Fasting and Exercise

Myths still exist that caution people away from getting involved in any type of exercise program or physical training during periods of intermittent fasting. Although it's true that your body will not perform well for an extended period of time on empty, but true intermittent fasting is not about complete deprivation. It is periodic, scheduled time away from food that lasts for mere hours.

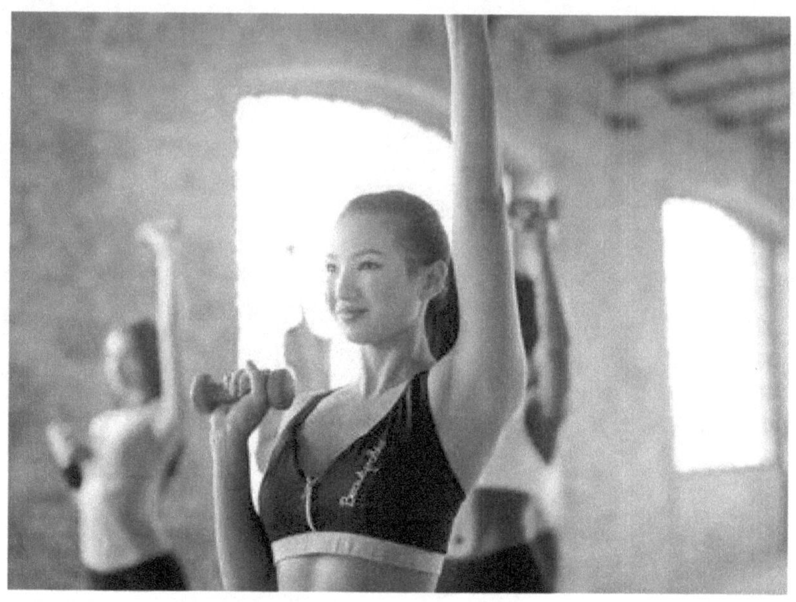

As long as you follow the correct methods for intermittent fasting and eat right during your window of nutritional opportunity, you can use exercise routines to increase the power output of your body. Running lean means a more efficient firing of your internal engine.

Optimizing the Eating Window and Exercise Routine Timing

If you are doing a slight exercise routine two or three days a week for general health maintenance, the timing between your physical exertion and eating is not as critical as for those that are trying to boost performance or build strength. A 30-minute to a 1-hour exercise program is less taxing on the body than the typical 2- or 3-hour workouts many athletes undergo.

2-Meal Daily Eating is Essential:

Muscle building and maintaining nutrients have to be replaced after your body pulls from reserves. You'll begin to experience weakness and a distinct loss in muscle tone by trying to continue strenuous physical fitness routines while only eating one meal per 24-hour period. Stick to a 2-meal regimen!

Optimal Eating Window:

The length of time considered the "window" between times of physical exercise routines and eating has been measured by a number of organizations that are too numerous to name. The determinations are that the premium response by the body in receiving post-exercise nutrition is between 1 and 3-hours. The benefits remain the same throughout this 3-hour period and drop off dramatically beyond the time limit.

You will need to adjust the time of your exercise routine to fit this window or move the time of your meal. An example is that starting your exercise at 6 am and finishing at 8 am would mean moving your lunch meal up to 10 or 11 am. You will have to move the evening meal up by the same amount of time to keep your intermittent fasting schedule on track.

Why the Intake of High-Density Foods is Important to Performance, Stamina, and Muscle Retention

Any type of regular exercise routines done during intermittent fasting periods will require that you fill up on high-density protein and carbohydrate-rich foods during your meals. The time you do this with casual exercise is not as critical as scheduled physical training designed to build, strengthen, and empower muscles.

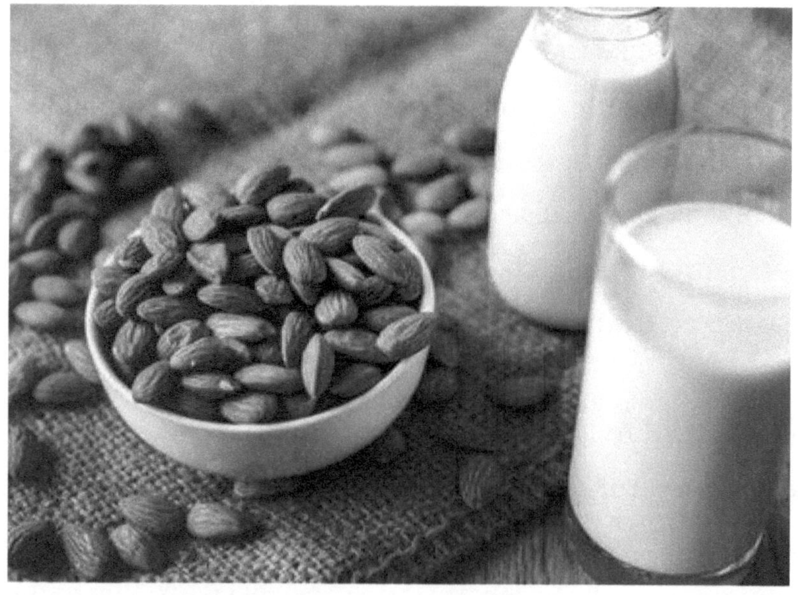

Muscle tissue is in the desired condition to grow and improve directly after an intense workout. Feeding yourself the proteins and carbohydrates necessary to accommodate this demand must happen during the 1 to 3-hour window directly following your physical exertion. Not following this natural ebb and flow of energy burn and refueling can cost you in stamina, muscle growth, and strength.

Take time to experiment with the best times to work out and follow-up with the needed nutrition. It might be easier to move your exercise time closer to the meals. It IS possible to maintain intermittent fasting schedules and stick with a rigorous exercise routine as long as you keep the type of nutrition in mind, time it well, and eat twice a day.

Transition Slowly

Think of your first month of intermittent fasting as an experiment, rather than a difficult task you must do in order to be healthy. Just relax and break it down into small, manageable tasks you know you can accomplish. When you're ready, consider increasing the number of days in the week that you fast for 14-hours, or consider fasting longer on the days of the week you choose to fast. See below for an example of how to build on the plan described above by adding a **15-hour fasting period** to your schedule. The first step is to complete:

<u>Day 1</u>: **Don't snack,** eat dinner at 7 pm, but no food after this meal for the day.

<u>Day 2</u>: **Put off breakfast until 10 AM.** You had dinner at 7 pm last night, no food before bed, and pushed off breakfast until 10 am. You just completed a 15-hour long fast – *and* you didn't eat a single snack! You are an intermittent fasting champion. Check in with how you are feeling, and make sure that you stop to enjoy your breakfast and lunch today. *After lunch on the second day, don't eat until dinner.* Dinner should be eaten at 7 pm. As with the prior steps: no snacks following dinner, serve breakfast at 10 am, and no between meal snacking.

Wait a day or two before repeating this schedule since it's your first time spending 15-hours in the **fasted** state. It takes patience but transitioning slowly is the best thing you can do for your health and the long-term success of intermittent fasting as a lifestyle approach. Don't rush it. Take the time to pay attention to any signals your body is sending you. If you are not feeling well, back off on the number of hours you are fasting between dinner and breakfast the next day, **but don't snack or eat small frequent meals.**

Do choose to have water, unsweetened tea or black coffee between meals. If you are feeling great, try this approach for a couple of weeks. Accomplishing the feat of staying in the **fasted** state a full 15-hours for just 2 times per week is a huge accomplishment! Take the time to do it right so you can progress at the pace that is right for you. In this way, you make it less likely to experience difficulties or unpleasant side effects. If you are feeling good following this approach for 1-2 weeks, it's safe to add in additional days during the week where you fast for a 15-hour period.

If you prefer an alternate day approach, you are ready to move to the next step: fasting for 16-18 hours. **Do not do this until you are ready.** This is only appropriate 1-2 months into intermittent fasting *after you have successfully fasted for 14 or 15-hour periods, 2-3 times per week.* If you have taken the first steps and are ready, go ahead and commit to a **16-18 hour fast,** 2-3 days per week. This means that the time between breakfast and dinner will increase for you up to a full 16-18 hours. Do not be tempted to start here. It's not appropriate to do this until you are ready as this amount of fasting time is not advised for women who are completely new to intermittent fasting.

<u>Day 1:</u> **Don't snack,** eat dinner at 6 pm, and don't eat at all after dinner. You can adjust the time of dinner to fit with your schedule and lifestyle, but since your goal is to wait 16-18

hours before eating again, eating earlier gives you more flexibility the next morning.

<u>Day 2</u>: Skip breakfast. If you had dinner at 6 pm last night, you need to wait at least until 12 noon before eating if your goal is to spend a full 16-hours in the **fasted** state. It's OK to skip breakfast, contrary to popular belief (more about this in Chapter 4). Drink water, tea, or coffee in the morning, and remind yourself that you can enjoy a wonderful meal at noon. That's just a few short hours away. If you have taken the time to transition slowly into the lifestyle of intermittent fasting by beginning with shorter fasting periods as recommended, you may find that this goal is easily accomplished without unpleasant hunger cravings. If you do not feel well, you are probably not ready to take this step. Pay attention, however, don't give yourself an easy out if your cravings are getting the best of you! Stop if you do not feel well, but otherwise, wait it out. You are so close to accomplishing your goal! If all is well, continue.

12:30-2 PM: Time to eat! Find a way to take a break and enjoy this meal if you possibly can. You may not be hungry but do eat at this point. Choose light nourishing foods such as soup, fresh grains, and vegetables to savor. Eat slowly and appreciate the meal. It's important to eat at this point for nutritional concerns, even if you don't feel you need to.

Spending time in the **fed** state is an important part of the balanced diet and lifestyle approach of intermittent fasting. The goal is to become free of your cravings, break unhealthy habits, and feel free to truly enjoy the food you eat. It's not about deprivation and hardship, so don't make it harder than it needs to be. Go ahead and eat and enjoy it as much as you possibly can without trying to extend the fasting period any more than 16-18 hours.

After lunch on the second day, don't eat until dinner. Have dinner at 7 pm, or when you are hungry. Remember not to snack, and to eat healthy food you enjoy when you choose to have your evening meal. Build on the prior steps: wait a day or two before trying to fast 16-18 hours again. When you are ready, repeat this program, but no more than 2-3 days total for the first week.

At this point, it may feel normal for you to spend anywhere from 12-15 hours between dinner and breakfast. The exact amount of time is not important. The important part is to remember not to eat after dinner and not to snack in between meals. By this point, you have probably become more attuned to your bodies needs and will be able to gauge what is the right time for you to eat breakfast. Remember to not skip it altogether more than 2-3 times the first week. The goal is to transition gradually, and this is accomplished by not increasing the window of time between dinner and breakfast too rapidly. The goal is a slow building upon the progress you have already made without upsetting the natural equilibrium of the body.

The best way to transition slowly is to build towards increasing the number of times when you spend 16-hours in the **fasted** state. The name for this protocol is the *16/8 method*. It has several variations in addition to the introductory approach described above. It's easy to do since many people aren't too hungry first thing in the morning. It can seem relatively painless to forego breakfast and reap all the benefits of intermittent fasting. This approach works because you reduce the time you spend in the **fed** state to an 8-hour window. You ultimately tip the scale towards spending ¾ of your day (16-hours) in the **fasted** state. **Using the 16/8 method is the best way to transition** to an intermittent fasting lifestyle for most women. Remember not to rush the process. This goal is most efficiently and safely achieved by taking the time to build on a natural 12-hour interval in the **fasted** state. There's no rush: be sure to take the steps that help you achieve your goals without compromising your health and wellbeing. Intermittent fasting is not about sacrifice and hardship so there is no need to force anything.

Learn to Listen to Your Body

Observe how your body responds and think about anything that comes up. The goal is learning from this process and finding a way to do it that works for you. If you start to feel hunger cravings or like you are depriving yourself without cause, return to the reasons why you decided to try intermittent fasting and revisit the benefits. It's a good idea to avoid snacks. Keep this principle at the front of your mind as you begin exploring how to incorporate intermittent fasting into your life. The goal is to eat consciously and that often means breaking old eating habits that no longer serve us.

Symptoms You Should Watch for

If you don't feel well, do not delay breakfast, even if it is the first time you are trying intermittent fasting. If you skipped dinner the night before, and wake up not feeling well, eat something simple. If you need to eat breakfast at 7 am, give yourself permission to do so this time. It's not a problem. That's 12-hours out of 24, and it's a fine place to start. All you had to do was get through the tough time after dinner, go to bed, and wake up. ***It's ideal to have an open and honest discussion with your physician before embarking on*** *the intermittent fasting diet. You should always heed their advice if you have any underlying medical conditions or take prescription medications. Certain medicines can interfere with the effectiveness of this diet regime. And, most importantly, if you are ill, or begin to feel sick, stop fasting.*

Chapter 4: How to Stay Motivated

Busting the Myths

- **Intermittent fasting will decrease metabolic rate.** Fasting is proven to increase your metabolic rate when done the right way. You will benefit from a leaner weight loss that helps retain the most muscle mass possible.

- **It is not OK to skip breakfast.** Contrary to popular belief, breakfast is not sacred or more important than any other meal. It is neutral. You can take it or leave it. Skipping breakfast won't add weight since you take in zero calories. Eating breakfast won't rev up the metabolic rate any more than another meal. So, go ahead and let go of the myth that you can't skip breakfast if this is what is holding you back.

- **You need to eat small meals throughout the day.** There is no basis to the belief that snacking boosts metabolism. Current research shows that snacking can contribute to fatty liver disease. It's perfectly fine and healthy to eat reasonably sized nutritious meals. Although widely accepted as a method of weight loss, there is no basis for the idea that eating multiple small meals throughout the day is a good strategy. It may serve the process of decreasing overall calorie consumption, but it's not a fast-track to weight loss. This eating pattern introduces a constant supply of calories and does not give the body time to recover and regenerate.

Common Intermittent Fasting Mistakes to Avoid

Tea and coffee don't count, but cream and sugar do!

Don't make the mistake of thinking added fats and sugars don't matter. If you choose to undertake intermittent fasting, follow the rules. Don't think that you can sneak some cream into your coffee or some sugar into your tea. If you want to do this, and you are ready to take a break from your fast for whatever reason, then treat yourself. Just don't call it a fasted period, because it isn't if your body is putting out the effort to process the fat or sugar consumed. Even small amounts will throw your system off and the metabolic process of your body will be altered. Any amount, no matter how small, of protein or carbohydrate will trigger your metabolism and begin the myriad processes put into effect once digestion is activated.

Once these processes begin, you are not fasting. Get used to drinking your tea plain and your coffee black while fasting.

Don't drink too much coffee.

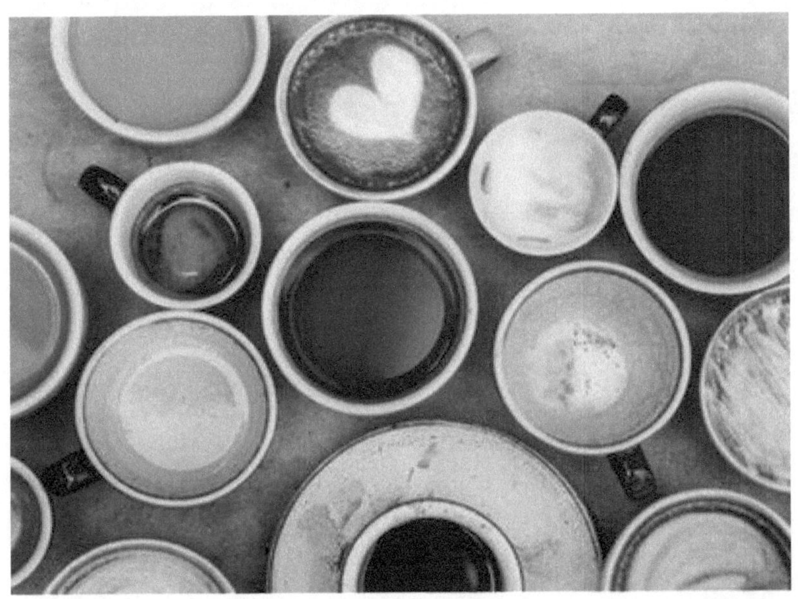

You guessed it, this was coming. Of course, whatever amount of coffee you decide is right for you must be black. Some women seem to fuel their lives on coffee. This may be fine, but be careful while you are fasting to observe if the way your body responds is different. Drinking Black coffee while fasting is somewhat controversial. Some people love it for its fat-burning effect, while others say that caffeine will set off your insulin response. Unfortunately, it has the impact of effectively taking you out of fasting mode. It's perfectly safe to drink black coffee during the fasting window, but be careful about how much. Make sure to compensate with extra water, because coffee deprives your system of fluids.

Coffee is considered a diuretic, which is a compound that causes your body to produce a ton of urine. Is it because caffeine increases blood flow through the kidneys? No one has honestly taken the time to find out and published studies. If you are not careful, your body can suffer from dehydration. It's less of a risk to drink coffee while you are eating because you actually receive large amounts of water from foods.

Caffeine is another question. Research indicates it can contribute to burning fat and suppress the appetite. That's all fine and good but don't consume so much that you get a buzz from it, as this may mean it triggers the insulin response you want to avoid while in the fasted state. Be careful with decaf as well. It still has diuretic properties and contains significantly more caffeine than black tea or green tea. The bottom line with coffee, regular or decaf, is that you do not want to become dehydrated.

Drink enough water.

Do not make the mistake of not drinking enough water! No matter how much coffee or tea you are drinking while fasting, you need to be sure to drink plenty of water. You'll hear a ton of different advice on the exact amount needed every day, but base it on your activity level. Decide what is right for you. It's commonly recommended that women try and consume eight, 8-ounce glasses, which equals about 2-liters, or a half a gallon of water in a 12-hour period. Keep in mind this is a minimum amount. Few studies indicate that you can drink too much water, so don't be afraid to drink more than you normally would.

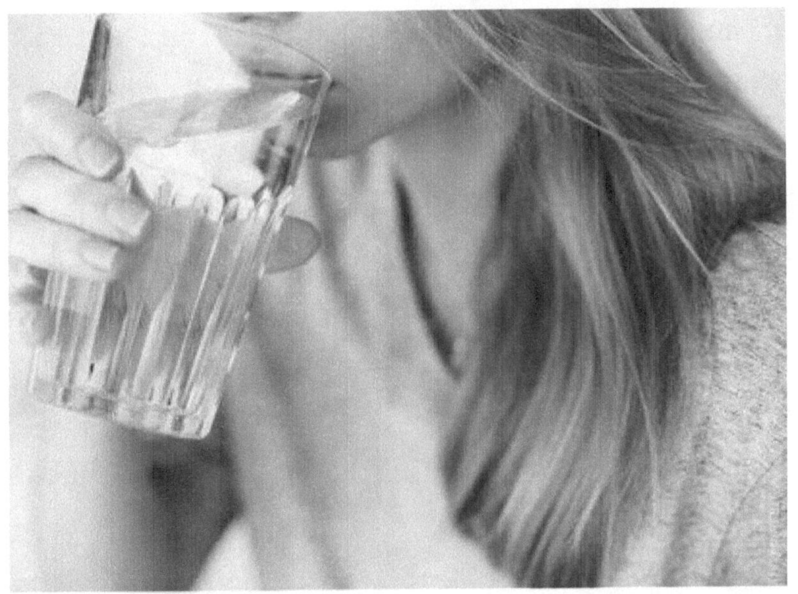

Remember that your body is not getting any water from food during the **fasted** state. It makes it more crucial you don't deprive your system of needed water. This is probably the single most fundamental part of intermittent fasting. It will not work without water. You cannot fast without drinking water. You can certainly also drink tea, and whatever amount of coffee you can handle, but don't forget to drink water. This is true of the time you spend in the **fed** state as well, but it's twice as important not to become dehydrated while fasting. All the cellular regeneration and rebuilding that is going on requires water. The waste products in your system that need to be released throughout the process of fasting require being flushed out, which calls for water.

If you make the mistake of not drinking water, you risk the possibility of becoming sick or having adverse symptoms including, but not limited to, headaches, nausea, lightheadedness or muscle pain. In summary, make sure to drink lots of water during your fasting window. It will serve the purpose of keeping you well-hydrated and help you detoxify at the same time. You can incorporate other no-calorie drinks as well, including herbal tea, apple cider vinegar, or mineral supplements. Start small and make sure any additives have zero calories and they don't upset your stomach. Be especially careful with mineral or vitamin supplements, as they can cause nausea while fasting.

Don't make the mistake of using intermittent fasting as an excuse to eat only unhealthy food.

Intermittent fasting offers many great health benefits and it would be a significant mistake to counter-act the benefits by choosing to eat only processed food. Intermittent fasting can help mitigate the effects of a bad diet, but it's not a reason to give yourself a free pass to go and eat all the junk you can lay your hands on.

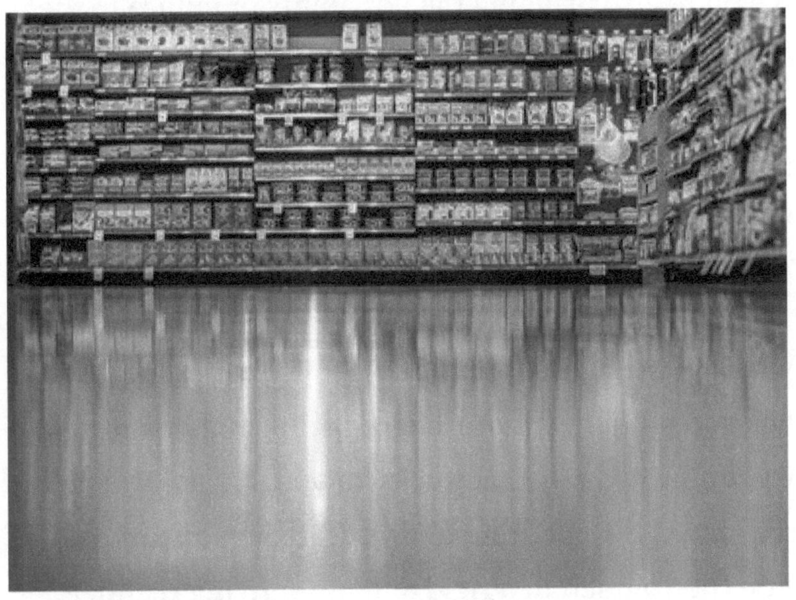

Intermittent fasting does help increase your metabolic flexibility and your ability to handle the occasional turkey dinner. It can even assist with occasional all you can eat buffet. Don't think it gives you a free pass to eat only junk food all the time. That's a sure recipe for disaster and not at all how intermittent fasting is intended to be used. It leads to even more bad eating habits, which is what you are trying to correct.

While intermittent fasting is a physical process, allowing our bodies the opportunity to repair and rejuvenate, it's also a mental exercise. It's a choice to fast we are making out of our own free will. When you try to be too militant or rigidly follow the clock, you're taking the choice away and inviting burnout. And, you're also bringing the possibility of failure to the table. If you normally don't eat until after 8 pm but you don't finish eating until 8:15, don't sweat the small stuff. The extra 15-minutes won't undo your efforts.

Fasting is also not the same as depriving ourselves of food. If you're hungry, famished and out of sorts, then eat! That may be what you need today and tomorrow you can try again to see if the process will go more smoothly. It's important that it fits into your life in a way that works for you. It's not worth forcing. Force makes it something to dread. It's not an area of life you want to tie yourself to a rigid and unforgiving regimen.

As you practice intermittent fasting more, to the point it becomes a part of your life, you'll start to learn the difference between the *ghrelin hormonal cycles of hunger* that pass easily and the very real need to eat. Don't push yourself too fast. Find a way to do it that works for you where you can forgive yourself, celebrate your successes and forgive your mistakes. The point is to become healthier and happier, not guilty because you've let yourself down.

Guilt never does anyone any good.

Don't try to be so strict about intermittent fasting that you take the fun and experimental joy out of the process. You'll be missing out on the best part. The key to success is to find the right fit for you, not to fit yourself to a rigid program.

Don't make the mistake of not eating enough during the eating window.

While intermittent fasting is effective and useful when practiced in conjunction with a weight loss goal, it's not, in and of itself, a diet. It's a mistake to use intermittent fasting as a form of purposeful, targeted calorie restriction. Intermittent fasting gives your body time to repair and clean out the cellular junk that's hanging around.

It leads to better function of all your body's systems, and it's important to support this with enough food to replenish and rebuild. Choose good, healthy, whole foods with lots of nutrient density and your body will get better at signaling when you have had enough. You will get better at listening to your body. You may find that you eat less than you did before, naturally, without having to be restrictive and regimented from the start.

Transition slowly

Once people are introduced to intermittent fasting and find out about how great it is with its many benefits, they are eager to dive in. Instead of easing in and slowly transitioning in a way that is right for their bodies, they dive straight in, trying for long 6 to 18-hour fasts. Don't make this mistake! It can lead to overwhelming hunger, frustration and a quick end to the trial of intermittent fasting.

Intermittent fasting is a powerful tool to help your body rest and repair that's been used throughout many cultures in human history. While it may be natural to the human body, it won't be natural to your body if you haven't spent a lifetime practicing the method. It can be a lifelong practice, but only if you give yourself time to adjust.

Top Fasting Hacks & Tips

Here are some strategies to help you get through the night:

- If you wake up hungry, drink water or a warm cup of unsweetened tea rather than automatically grabbing a snack. Remind yourself why you are fasting!
- Brush your teeth, use mouthwash, and floss. The minty taste of toothpaste and the clean feeling can help curb cravings. The act of brushing your teeth also can signify

that you're done eating for the day: most of us do not want to have to brush our teeth twice! Just this small act can be enough to get your mind on a different track that isn't focused on food.

- Sleep through the cravings. It's okay because you had plenty of food to eat during the day and you ate a good dinner. If you can't sleep, distract yourself with a good book or a magazine. Try not to use your phone, tablet or computer at night. You will reap the most benefits from fasting if you are in a relaxed, calm and restful state.

Here are some tips to help you avoid snacking:

- When you want something to eat, drink a non-caloric drink instead.
- Dinner will be in a very short amount of time. You can make it for a few hours! Remind yourself that you will get to eat soon and that you will enjoy it even more because you have built up anticipation. You just need to practice patience and wait.
- Stay busy. Get some work done, make a phone call, pursue a hobby you enjoy and need to make time for, or take on a task you need to complete.

- Hunger pains come in waves that are temporary and fleeting. They do not get worse with time: you can count on the fact that they will subside. Wait them out.

- Remind yourself that your hunger may be your mind playing tricks on you. You may be thirsty, or just craving a snack because it's a certain time of day, or a certain thing is happening. Remember, you are trying to change your habits. Take control of the situation and check in to see what you are thinking or feeling. Look for the easy solutions, such a grabbing a glass of water. Snacking habits can be hard to break. Experiencing stress, anxiety, or even boredom can trigger the compulsion to eat.

Here is an approach that allows you to make intermittent fasting normal and fun:

- Repetition is the best way to make intermittent fasting second nature. Keep it up! Just remember to proceed at a pace that is appropriate for you.

- Practice *mindful eating* while you are fasting and remember to engage in another activity that keeps your mind off food and eating.

- Always remember hunger is fleeting and short-lived. Learn the ways that work for *you* to help you ride out your hunger waves until they go away. Always remember that you are much stronger than any of your cravings.

- Avoid eating for any other reason than getting necessary nutrition. Wait to eat until you *truly* felt hungry. This knowledge will come in time as a result of practice. Be patient!

Conclusion

Thank you for making it through to the end of <u>Intermittent Fasting for Women.</u>

We hope it was informative and able to provide you with all the tools you need to achieve your goals, whatever they may be. There is so much more to learn about your health and your body than this book can contain. We sincerely hope this is only the beginning of your journey towards self-discovery, weight management, and optimum health.

The next step is to decide the right approach to intermittent fasting for you and your unique life situation. You now have the background and the knowledge needed to evaluate how intermittent fasting works and how this process can benefit you and your health.

The first step is to evaluate your eating habits and observe how food makes you feel. Pay close attention to everything you eat and how it affects your emotions. Consider writing it down and building times into your day where you can appreciate your meals and how food provides the energy your body needs. Pay attention to what, when, and how you eat. When you're ready, start experimenting by spending one day without eating after dinner. Next, try skipping snacks during the day.

Once completing this initial trial of self-observation and conscious eating behavior, you may find that you're ready to try an intermittent fast. Avoid making the common mistakes covered in this book and you'll be well on your way to enjoying the benefits of regular intermittent fasting without health complications.

Please take the necessary steps to start intermittent fasting slowly, but don't be afraid to commit and be diligent if you're ready. Remember to be patient with yourself and enjoy the process. Intermittent fasting is a journey, not a regimen. You'll be most successful if you work with your body, rather than fight a battle within. The beauty of intermittent fasting is that you can make it work for you, rather than needing to conform to a rigid plan. Thank you for reading, and we hope you will enjoy the journey ahead, in whatever way it unfolds for you!

Finally, if you found this book useful in any way, a review on Amazon is always appreciated!

Free Bonuses

Go to link <u>http://bit.ly/IFfreebonuses</u> **and you will get**

1. **Printable 7 Day Food Journal** to have an accurate picture of your dietary habits
2. **5 keys** to a healthy diet for you and your family
3. **Free E-Book About Eating Real Foods** to accelerate your journey towards optimum health and weight from today

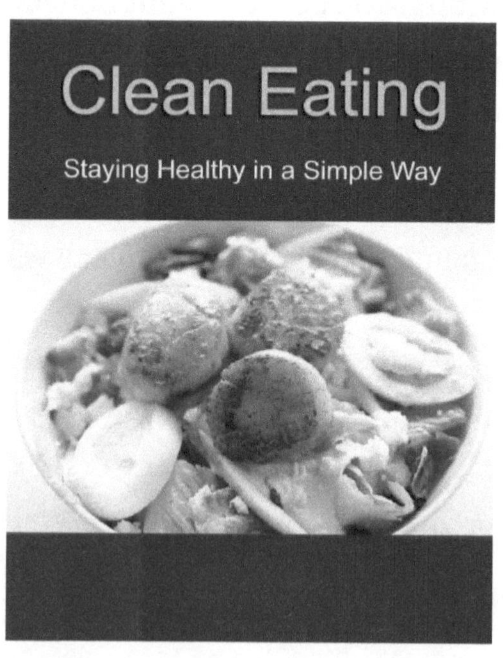

Download the Audio Book Version of This Book for FREE

If you love listening to audio books on-the-go, I have great news for you. You can download the audio book version of this book for **FREE** just by signing up for a **FREE** 30-day audible trial! See below for more details!

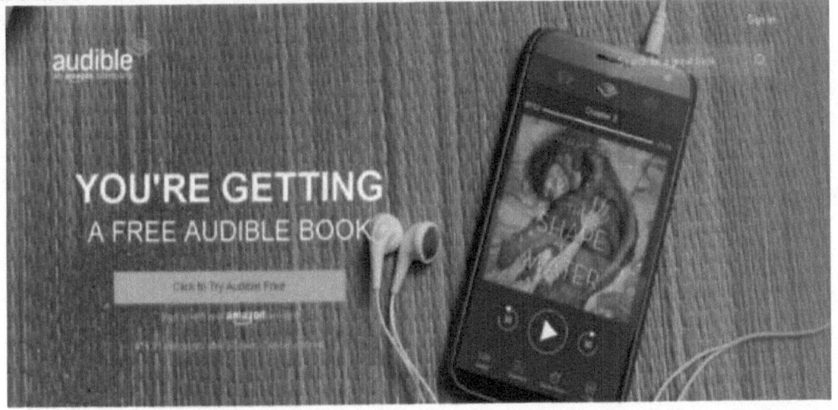

Audible **FREE** 30 day Trial Benefits

- **3 x FREE audible titles** (this book + 2 Audible Originals)

- Listen **anywhere** with the Audible app across multiple devices

- Cancel anytime and **keep all your audiobooks**

- After trial **3 x FREE audible titles** each month

- Choose from Audible's **200,000 +** Titles

- Roll over any unused credits for **up to 5 months**

- Make **easy, no-hassle exchange** of any audiobook you don't love

- **Exclusive** audio-guided wellness programs

Go to the links below to get started!

For Audible US: https://adbl.co/2XFw2Ez

For Audible UK: https://adbl.co/2UlAEOf

For Audible FR: http://bit.ly/2tSMfZo

For Audible DE: https://adbl.co/2UkHCTn